What if it's

Migraine Treatments and Remedies

Skinny Book™

By:

Sarah E. Maggiore BSN (C), RN (C)
With Dr. Jack Maggiore

Table of Contents

ABOUT THE AUTHOR – SARAH MAGGIORE

For as long as I could remember, most of my days have been intruded by a pain in my head. Sometimes the pain greets me as I awake in bed, and sometimes it gives me the benefit of letting me know that it's on its way. Even before I was able to communicate to my parents that my head hurt, my face and temperament spoke for me. Photographs have captured in my face what was most certainly a headache in my miniscule two-year-old body. And when my ornery mannerisms weren't enough to let my family know I was hurting, nausea would kick in to put the exclamation point on an otherwise predictable day for me. Yes, migraine has always been a part of my life, and while I absolutely hate to personify this villain who has stolen my childhood, has shaped my personality, and has made every week of my life miserably challenging, I recognize that I am not alone. Even among my family, I share this trait with my father, two of my four siblings, and a number of cousins, all of whom are intelligent and inherent overachievers in every aspect of the word. I often wonder how much more we could accomplish if we weren't limited by migraine.

My need to find answers to medical dilemmas like migraine was actually one of the reasons I chose a career in a health care profession. Nursing was my calling – as the need to be involved in patient interactions, serving as an advocate, an educator, a liaison, and voice, weighed heavily in my decision. With just weeks remaining before graduation at St. Ambrose University and receiving my bachelor 's degree in nursing, I am proud to share with you my life's experiences and personal research with migraine. To assist me in providing a clinical rationale for the causes and treatments of migraine, I have sought the expertise of my father, fellow migraine sufferer, Dr. Jack Maggiore, a doctoral clinical pathologist who specializes in the understanding of the process of diseases. As a clinical diagnostician, Dr. Maggiore has always been bothered that the diagnosis of migraine has been one of exclusion of other causes for headaches. Our collective desire is to provide you with a resource that provides you with more answers than questions. If our migraine references allow you to spend just one day free from the debilitating pain of a headache, we know you will have invested your time wisely in realizing the value of a headache-free day.

Sarah Eileen Maggiore, BSN (C), RN (C)

January 30, 2012

PREFACE

For those of us, the unfortunate millions who are susceptible to migraine headaches, our search for pain relief may be the single most important need to our wellbeing. Before jumping right into an overview of the remedies and treatments, you need to know that the onset of a migraine headache most likely occurs from a chain reaction of three distinct events. First, there is a rise in blood pressure, of which there are many causes and triggers. Second, an opening of the blood vessels in the brain and head occurs in an attempt to reduce the blood pressure. This is called vasodilation, which literally means "veins open". Third, pain in the head results from the increased blood flow and inflammation in the area. Blood pressure increases, blood vessels open wider in the head, and pain occurs from the inflammation and blood flow to the sensitive tissues in the head. That provides the basis for the treatments and remedies discussed in this book, as one or more of these mechanisms is being addressed in an attempt to reduce the debilitation that is being experienced with a migraine headache.

Chapter 1

Over the Counter (OTC) Treatments

Ibuprofen

Brand Names	How it Works	What it Doesn't Do	Side Effects?
Motrin®, Advil®, Nuprin®	Anti-Inflammatory, Pain-Reliever, Fever-Reducer	Reduce blood pressure; Constrict dilated blood vessels	Yes: Decreases appetite, nausea, vomiting, heartburn, inflammation of the stomach lining

Ibuprofen is commonly known as Advil®, Motrin®, Motrin IB®, or Nuprin® and is widely available in generic and store brands. Ibuprofen is seen as an affordable remedy, and is widely used to treat and relieve a variety of general ailments. It is considered a Non-Steroidal Anti-inflammatory Drug, or NSAID. Ibuprofen has three main functions or intended uses: 1) it is an anti-inflammatory used to reduce swelling; 2) it is an antipyretic used to reduce fever; and 3) it is an analgesic used to reduce pain. Pain, inflammation, and fever result from the breakdown of naturally occurring chemicals in your body called prostaglandins [prah-stah-GLAN-dinz], which the body produces as part of the healing process. NSAID medications like ibuprofen inhibit prostaglandin synthesis. This means that taking an NSAID will help to interrupt the signal of pain that is intended to be received by brain. By taking ibuprofen, the pain of the migraine can be controlled and better tolerated so the migraine does not leave you debilitated. Simply stated, ibuprofen will take the edge off of the pain, but it does not eliminate it. Ibuprofen also does not have an action to reduce blood pressure nor constrict the blood vessels in the brain. While ibuprofen is generally well tolerated by children, adults, and seniors, there are some downsides to taking an NSAID too frequently or taking more than the recommended dose of the medication. Some of these negative effects are causing a decreased appetite, nausea, vomiting, heartburn, or inflammation of the lining of the stomach. As with all over-the-counter remedies, you must weigh the risk versus the benefit. If the relief obtained from taking the medication outweighs the side effects and long-term dangers, then it becomes a go-to option in your arsenal of choices to combat your migraine headaches. For many with migraines, any potential solution that provides a perceived measure of relief is to be considered and will remain on your treatment list unless the consequences are grave. If you have severe kidney disease or liver disease, asthma, a peptic ulcer, or are in the third trimester of pregnancy, you should not take NSAID medications, regardless of how effective they are at providing you with pain relief for your migraine headache.

Naproxen Sodium

Brand Names	How it Works	What it Doesn't Do	Side Effects?
Aleve®, Anaprox®, Naprosen®	Anti-Inflammatory, Pain-Reliever, Fever-Reducer	Reduce blood pressure; Constrict dilated blood vessels	Yes: Constipation, diarrhea, dizziness, lightheadedness, cold-like symptoms

Naproxen sodium, commonly known as Aleve®, Anaprox® or Naprosen®, is an NSAID like ibuprofen, and is taken to relieve pain, inflammation, and fever. Like ibuprofen, naproxen sodium will interrupt the pain that occurs with prostaglandin synthesis, and relief should be realized about 30 minutes after you take it. Naproxen sodium is typically more concentrated than ibuprofen, therefore the usual dose of 220 milligrams (mg) should be taken every 8-12 hours as needed for pain, rather than the 4-6 hours recommended for ibuprofen. Aside from the convenience of fewer doses needed per day, some women prefer naproxen sodium over ibuprofen for its ability to relieve menstrual pain and cramping, especially when migraine headaches tend to occur in conjunction with menstrual cycles. Naproxen sodium should be taken with food to prevent stomach upset, as the higher concentration of NSAID tends to cause stomach and intestinal discomfort when taken on an empty stomach. It is important to not take Naproxen sodium in conjunction with ibuprofen, other pain relievers, other over-the-counter medications, or certain cold medications because the content of these drugs are similar and can have harmful effects upon your kidneys and liver. Like all other drugs, it is important to follow the recommendation of the doctor for how to take the drug safely and effectively. Taking naproxen sodium regularly can cause constipation, diarrhea, dizziness and lightheadedness, and cold-like symptoms. It is important to call a doctor if you experience ringing in your ears, hearing problems, changes in your vision, pain in your upper stomach, new swelling, pain, redness, yellowing of your eyes or skin, back pain or pain while urinating, or an unusually fast heartbeat, as these are all indications of the negative side effects of the medication.

Acetaminophen

Brand Names	How it Works	What it Doesn't Do	Side Effects?
Tylenol®	Pain-Reliever, Fever-Reducer	Reduce blood pressure; Constrict dilated blood vessels	Yes: Decreases appetite, nausea, vomiting, low blood sugar, skin rash

Although I have never taken Tylenol® or any generic form of acetaminophen with the sole purpose to relieve the pain from my migraine headaches, it can be an effective option to treat migraine pain. Acetaminophen also inhibits prostaglandin synthesis and therefore is able to lessen severe pain. While acetaminophen is a commonly recommended and highly sought pain reliever, it does not have the anti-platelet or anti-inflammatory effects of aspirin or ibuprofen. Because of this, it is safe to take during pregnancy, however it should not be taken if you have liver disease, are malnourished, or an alcoholic, as acetaminophen is metabolized or broken down in the liver and requires a healthy liver to be properly metabolized and safely eliminated from the body. Common side effects from acetaminophen are loss of appetite, nausea, vomiting, low blood sugar, and a rash. Like all over-the-counter pain relievers, acetaminophen should be taken as recommended to ensure safety. Because acetaminophen and ibuprofen are both analgesics, but do not have other similar properties, the two medications can be alternated at two hour intervals to better control pain. You should always consult a physician before starting such a drug regimen, and whenever the pain becomes worse or lasts for more than 24 hours.

Aspirin

Brand Names	How it Works	What it Doesn't Do	Side Effects?
Bayer® Anacin®	Anti-Inflammatory, Pain-Reliever, Fever-Reducer, Anti-platelet	Reduce blood pressure; Constrict dilated blood vessels	Yes: Stomach discomfort, prolonged bleeding

Aspirin is included in the NSAID category of drugs. That means that it has analgesic, pain relieving properties. Aspirin also has anti-platelet effects, which means that it results in prolonged bleeding, should an injury occur to a blood vessel or tissues that are rich with a blood supply. For those who are already prescribed a low daily dose (such as 81 mg) of aspirin or baby aspirin to reduce the risk of heart attack and stroke, be mindful that turning to higher doses for purposes of pain relief may place you into a higher-than-recommended dose category for the purpose of preventing heart attacks and strokes. Consult your doctor or pharmacist for their recommendation on how to best manage preventive care with pain treatment. They may suggest forgoing your dose of baby aspirin to enable the high aspirin dose for pain relief. While some people report success with a simple aspirin in controlling the pain of a migraine headache, most find that aspirin used in combined therapies with acetaminophen and caffeine offers greater extended relief. See the next section.

Combined Analgesics with Caffeine — Excedrin®

Brand Names	How it Works	What it Doesn't Do	Side Effects?
Excedrin®	Anti-Inflammatory, Pain-Reliever, Fever-Reducer, Constrict dilated blood vessels, Accelerates Medicine Uptake	Reduce blood pressure	Yes: Nervousness, jittery, Increases heart rate, stomach discomfort, prolonged bleeding

Excedrin, especially when combined with sleeping, seems to be the best remedy to help me get over my migraine headaches. Excedrin is composed of 250 mg of acetaminophen, 250 mg of aspirin, and 65 mg of caffeine. Acetaminophen acts as a pain reliever and fever reducer. Aspirin is also a fever reducer and pain reliever, in addition to having properties as an anti-inflammatory agent, and anti-platelet agent which is used to prevent blood clots. The caffeine is used because it has the ability to speed up the drug delivery to the tissues, and also functions to constrict the blood vessels. Vasoconstriction is the narrowing of smooth muscle of the blood vessel walls by constricting. This can be likened to squeezing the outside of a drinking straw. So why is this a good thing? Remember that the pain of migraine headaches is thought to be caused by the dilation or the opening of the blood vessels. The dose of caffeine in Excedrin acts to assist controlling the pain by decreasing the size of the vessels and reducing the excessive blood flow to the head. This occurs while the acetaminophen and aspirin work together to help control the pain and inflammation of the blood vessels and surrounding tissues. Because Excedrin has as much caffeine as one cup of coffee, some who take it feel nervousness, jittery, restless, and experience an increase in heart rate. Some people report nausea, as with any aspirin-containing medications. Excedrin should not be given to children under the age of 12 because of the adverse effects that can occur from aspirin. If Excedrin is not taken as recommended or is taken daily as a preventative agent for migraine headaches, liver, kidney, and stomach lining damage can occur. Excedrin should not be taken with other NSAID medication or other aspirin-containing treatment because it can cause a negative effect on the body. If you are pregnant you should not take Excedrin to treat your migraine because caffeine and aspirin are not recommended for consumption during pregnancy and could have harmful effects on the placenta and bloodstream of the baby.

Chapter 2

Natural Remedies

For those who seek to limit the ingestion or use of chemical means to relieve migraine headaches, there are many available natural and nutraceutical means of relieving and possibly preventing migraine headaches. Nutraceutical is a term that is used to indicate a product that is isolated or purified from a naturally occurring substance that has a positive physiological benefit. As a disclaimer, unless otherwise indicated, the benefits of these remedies have not been reviewed or approved by the FDA as being specific in treating migraine headaches. Where possible, an explanation as to a purported or theoretical mechanism is provided. Further, be sure to talk to your health care provider before starting to take herbs or supplements as a treatment for migraines, as many of these treatments, although available over-the-counter, have side effects and may interact with other prescribed medications.

Magnesium

How it Works	What it Doesn't Do	Side Effects?
Regulates muscle contractions and nerve impulses, reduces blood pressure	Relieve pain	Yes. Diarrhea, stomach irritation, low blood pressure

Vitamin B-Complex

How it Works	What it Doesn't Do	Side Effects?
Regulates reactions in the body that produce serotonin, a chemical that regulates blood vessel constriction	Relieve pain, Reduce blood pressure	Yes. May cause dark or orange-tinged urine, which is not clinically significant

On a personal note, my father, a life-long migraine sufferer, told me that he sought the guidance of a neurologist to manage his headaches. His neurologist suggested that the available body of research supported daily dietary supplementation with 400 mg of magnesium and a vitamin B-50 complex tablet to control the frequency and intensity of his migraine headaches. My father is a clinical pathologist and is highly evidence-based in his approach to medicine. That means that he relies upon strong scientific evidence through clinical trials with well-designed study protocols before consenting to the belief of a treatment benefit. As you could imagine, he was skeptical that somebody could experience a benefit from supplementing a diet with vitamins and minerals. Knowing this about my father, his neurologist provided him with a mini library of published references on the benefits of B-vitamins and magnesium. Prior to this therapy, my father experienced migraine headaches 2-3 times per week since age 5. Sometimes his headaches lasted 3 days and twice had resulted in temporary loss of vision in his left eye. Missed work and lack of productivity when he had migraine headaches were common for him, and he turned to Excedrin as his primary OTC remedy. Within a week of using the supplements, my father recalls not needing to seek the relief of the Excedrin that he keeps in constant supply in the top drawer of his desk, glove compartment, and outside pouch of his computer case, as he never knew when and where a migraine headache would come on like a raging bull. He shared with me his migraine diary, a calendar of the frequency and duration of his headaches. Now five years later, what was once a near daily headache occurrence has been reduced to once or twice per month. What were headaches that lasted for days are now headaches that are gone within hours.

Because I was desperate for a solution to my migraines, I tried the remedy as well. Taking one magnesium supplement (250 mg of Magnesium oxide tablet) and one B-50 complex vitamin each morning decreased the frequency of my migraine headaches. It is important to take the recommended amount of magnesium per day because magnesium is a mineral that is involved in regulating muscle contractions and nerve impulses. Magnesium should be taken on an empty stomach to increase its absorption and avoid the formation of less active forms as it combines with other substances in the diet. Aside from the tablet forms of magnesium widely available wherever vitamins are sold, magnesium is also found naturally in beans, grains, vegetables, seeds, and nuts, as well as in dairy products, fish, meats, chocolate and coffee. Adult males are suggested to intake 400-420 mg per day and women are suggested to intake 310-320 mg per day. When the necessary amount is not consumed in the diet, normal muscle and nerve function is impaired. You may notice your muscles twitching.   Magnesium supplements help to regulate muscle contractions, which assist in relieving the rapid contraction and dilation of the vessels in the brain that cause the pain of the migraine headache. Magnesium is also taken to decrease the risk of high blood pressure. Consistent high blood pressure in the vessels in your head will contribute to the tendency for the blood vessels to dilate in an attempt to relieve the blood pressure. Both of these mechanisms result in the head pain that is experienced as a migraine headache. Most neurological and headache experts agree that magnesium is a safe and inexpensive option to be considered to help prevent the onset of migraine headaches, as well as reduce their frequency and intensity. Too high of a dose of magnesium may result in diarrhea and stomach irritation, as well as causing low blood pressure. Magnesium may also counteract the benefits of supplements taken to treat osteoporosis, so check with your doctor before self-medicating.

Taking B- complex vitamins serves to help with the regular functioning of the nervous system and converting food to energy. Vitamin B-complex also regulates chemical reactions that occur within the body and promotes the production of serotonin [sair-o-TONE-in]. The exact function of serotonin in the body is not fully understood. It is known, however, that it is a chemical used to relay messages between the nerve cells as well as regulating the constriction and dilation of the blood vessels in the brain. Decreased levels of serotonin are associated with the blood vessels in the brain dilating causing a migraine headache. More information about the role that serotonin plays upon migraines will be discussed further in the *What If It's... Migraines* book, available through Portrait Health Publishing.

Chai Tea

How it Works	What it Doesn't Do	Side Effects?
Contains ginger root which is anti-inflammatory	Relieve pain, Reduce blood pressure	None

It has long been told that drinking a warm cup of a ginger-rich tea such as Chai Tea can help prevent migraines. Chai Tea is a blended mix of spices and teas concocted from ginger root, cinnamon, cloves, cardamom, black peppercorn, fennel, with black or green tea leaves. Ginger has anti-inflammatory properties which may work to reduce the inflammation of the blood vessels in the brain. Chai tea also provides a reduced caffeine content which, if you have been told to reduce your caffeine intake as a potential migraine trigger, provides the comfort of tea, minus the stimulation of caffeine.

Feverfew

How it Works	What it Doesn't Do	Side Effects?
Contains parthenolide, which is anti-inflammatory and relieves smooth muscle spasms in dilated blood vessels.	Reduce blood pressure	Yes. Abdominal pain, gas, diarrhea, nausea, vomiting, nervousness, increases bleeding time, allergic reactions

Among the more widely publicized herbal remedies to treat migraine is an herbal plant called feverfew, which is readily available without a prescription at vitamin stores, nutrition outlets, and health food shops. The herb feverfew (*Tanacetum parthenium*) has been used for centuries in Europe as a remedy for headache, arthritis, pain, and fever. In one study to evaluate the effectiveness of feverfew as a preventive agent for migraine headaches, 170 people with chronic migraines were given either feverfew or a placebo sugar pill. Those who took feverfew had an average decrease in the number of migraine headaches by 1.9 per month, compared to the placebo, which decreased by 1.3 migraine headaches per month. While some have reported success with feverfew to prevent headaches, a more critical review of five studies on feverfew and migraines, involving a total of 343 people, concluded that results were mixed and did not convincingly establish that feverfew was effective for preventing migraine headaches.

The migraine-relieving activity of feverfew is believed to be due to parthenolide (par-THEN-o-lyd), an active compound it contains that helps relieve smooth muscle spasms. Specifically, it helps prevent the constriction of blood vessels in the brain. Parthenolide also inhibits the actions of compounds that cause inflammation.

Side effects of feverfew are numerous and may include abdominal pain, gas, diarrhea, nausea, vomiting, and nervousness. Feverfew is an extract of a weed-like plant, of which many people have allergies. People with allergies to chamomile, ragweed, or yarrow should not take feverfew. Feverfew may also increase bleeding time, so it should not be taken by people with bleeding disorders or blood clotting deficiencies. Feverfew may interact with "blood-thinning" medications, such as aspirin and warfarin (Coumadin®) and medications containing NSAIDs. People taking these medications should consult a healthcare practitioner before taking feverfew. The safety of feverfew in pregnant or nursing women or children has not been established.

Butterbur

How it Works	What it Doesn't Do	Side Effects?
Anti-inflammatory, Anti-spasmodic, Muscle Relaxant	Reduce blood pressure	Yes. Mild digestive complaints, fatigue, nausea, vomiting, diarrhea, constipation, allergic reactions

The herb butterbur (*Petasites hybridus*) is a shrub-like plant that grows in Europe and parts of Asia and North America. Butterbur is also widely available in nutrition and vitamin stores. Extracts made from the herb are used to treat migraine headaches, stomach cramps, coughs, allergies, and asthma. Several studies suggest that butterbur helps to prevent migraines. The largest study involved 245 people with migraines who took either butterbur extract (50 or 75 mg twice a day) or a placebo. After four months of treatment, butterbur, 75 mg twice a day but not 50 mg twice a day, was more effective than a placebo for migraines. Side effects were minor and included mild digestive complaints, fatigue, nausea, vomiting, diarrhea, and constipation. Pregnant or nursing women, children, or people with kidney or liver disease should not take butterbur.

Butterbur is in the ragweed plant family, so people who are allergic to ragweed, marigold, daisy, or chrysanthemum should not use butterbur. The raw herb as well as teas, extracts, and capsules made from the raw herb should not be used because they contain substances that can be toxic to the liver and kidneys and may cause cancer.

Griffonia

How it Works	What it Doesn't Do	Side Effects?
Rich in 5-HTP which the body converts to serotonin, a chemical that regulates blood vessel constriction	Reduce blood pressure	Yes. Decreases appetite , gas, nausea, stomach cramps, heartburn, nightmares, decreases sex drive

Griffonia is made from the seeds of as plant that is grown in Africa (*Griffonia simplicifolia*). It is commercially available at vitamin and nutrition stores under the name Natrol®. Griffonia is rich in a chemical substance called 5-HTP (5-Hydroxytryptophan). This substance is also naturally produced in the body from the amino acid tryptophan, which is found in the proteins that we consume. The body converts 5-HTP to the neurotransmitter serotonin and the hormone melatonin.

As a migraine reliever, research indicates that 5-HTP may prevent migraines and reduce the frequency and severity of migraine headaches. However, large randomized controlled trials are needed to confirm its effectiveness. In one study, 124 people were given 5-HTP (600 mg/day) or the prescription drug methysergide. After six months, 5-HTP was found to be as effective as methysergide, a prescription vasoconstrictor, in reducing the severity and duration of migraines.

Another study looked at 5-HTP and the drug propranolol for 4 months. Both treatments resulted in a statistically significant reduction in the frequency of migraines. However, the propranolol group fared better, with a reduction in the duration of episodes and the number of analgesics used for the treatment of episodes.

Many prescription treatments for migraine (see below) rely upon the same action on the receptors of serotonin. As with ANY supplement, consult your doctor before taking, even though these are readily available in nutrition and health food stores without a prescription.

Chapter 3

Prescription Treatments

Opioid and Narcotic Analgesics

Common Names and Brand Names	How it Works	What it Doesn't Do	Side Effects?
Codeine Fiorinal® Meperidine with Demerol®, Butorphanol®	Pain-Reliever	Reduce blood pressure; Constrict dilated blood vessels	Yes: Addictive narcotic Decreases appetite, nausea, respiratory distress

Opioid analgesics, such as codeine formulations may be prescribed to alleviate severe pain caused by migraines. These pain relievers interrupt the pain impulse at the spinal cord level. Because addiction to this medication is quite possible, those who have addictive tendencies should try not to use this as a form of pain relief. Feelings of nausea or decreased appetite often occur while taking opioid medications. Relief from pain should be felt within 1-2 hours of taking the medication. Because opioid analgesics are highly concentrated with pain relievers, prescriptions from your health care provider are necessary to obtain the medication. Your provider will instruct you on the proper regimen for taking opioid analgesics safely. This class of medications is not specific for migraine, but as a last resort when head pain is severe, prolonged and debilitating, your doctor may suggest a drug from this class.

Fiorinal® is a combination of aspirin, butalbital [byoo-TAL-buh- tal], and caffeine. This medication has been proven to be effective in treating tension headaches; a category of headaches similar to migraines which will be discussed more fully in the book, *What If It's... Migraines?*™, available through Portrait Health Publishing. A common form of this drug is Fiorinal with Codeine, which also requires a physician's prescription to obtain the medication.

Other opioid analgesics that have been used to treat migraines successfully are Meperidine with Demerol® and Butorphanol®. Butorphanol is usually prescribed as a nasal spray used to relieve pain. When inhaled through the nose, you are able to feel the effects of this medication within the first few minutes of inhalation and will last for approximately 2 to 4 hours. These medications should be taken with great caution because if the medication is not taken properly or the medication is abused, respiratory depression may occur with devastating results.

Ergot alkaloids (ergotamine tartrate):

Common Names and Brand Names	How it Works	What it Doesn't Do	Side Effects?
Cafergot® Ergostat® Migranal®	Enhances constriction of blood vessels	Reduce blood pressure	Yes: Abdominal cramping, nausea, vomiting, confusion

Ergot alkaloids, also known as ergotamine [air-GO-tah-meen] tartrate, are prescribed to reduce the blood flow to the head by enhancing constriction of the blood vessels. Because ergotamine is absorbed poorly through the digestive system, it needs to be taken as a tablet to be dissolved under your tongue, or inhaled, or used as a rectal suppository. An injectable form is also available to treat severe migraine cases, especially when a headache presents as a cluster-type headache. Ergotamine can be prescribed with caffeine to increase its absorption and its vasoconstrictive properties. Like all vasoconstrictive classes of drugs, this drug is potentially harmful to those who have a disease of the circulatory system, such as peripheral vascular disease, peripheral artery disease, atherosclerosis, or high blood pressure. Ergot alkaloids should also be avoided by those with anemia, liver or kidney disease, and especially in those who are pregnant because it can cause the muscles of the uterus to contract. Common side effects from taking ergot alkaloids are abdominal cramping, nausea and vomiting, and confusion. To increase the benefit of this drug, it is suggested that you take the medication as soon as the symptoms of a migraine headache occur and lay in a dark quiet room for 2 hours after taking the drug. This makes it a less-than-optimal choice for a workplace migraine treatment, although its success as a treatment is considered quick and effective.

Common drugs in this class are Cafergot® (with caffeine) and Ergostat®. Cafergot is used as a vasoconstrictor and the caffeine in its formulation is able to increase absorption of the medication into the blood stream. Ergostat is an alpha- adrenergic blocker and a vasoconstrictor that acts to help reduce the extra blood flow that is increased to your brain during a migraine. Dihydroergotamine [dy-HY-droh-air-GO-tah-meen] is a class of drug that is designed to be used solely for the relief of migraines and vascular headaches. It works by constricting the smooth muscle tissue of the blood vessels in the brain and blocks the release of serotonin which is a factor in causing migraines. It is best absorbed when administered through injections. Dihydroergotamines should absolutely not be taken if you are pregnant, have coronary artery disease, hypertension, Raynaud's phenomenon, peripheral vascular disease, angina, a history of heart attacks or stroke, Buerger's disease, or other cardiac diseases. Dihydroergotamines is commercially available as Migranal®, which may be prescribed as a self-injection.

Methysergide

Common Names and Brand Names	How it Works	What it Doesn't Do	Side Effects?
Sansert®	Narrows blood vessels in the head	Reduce blood pressure	Yes: Hallucinations

Methysergide [meth-uh-SER- jide] was first available in 1962, and is believed to act by narrowing the blood vessels that supply blood to the head. This prescription-use-only vasoconstrictive drug is used primarily to prevent vascular headaches and migraine headaches. One drug in this class is called Sansert®. It is rarely used in the United States, as one of its side effects is hallucinations, as it is very similar in chemical structure to LSD.

Selective serotonin (5-HT) receptor agonists or *Triptans*

Names	How it Works	Side Effects?
See table below for the *triptan* drug generic and brand names	Blocks serotonin receptors to reduce cranial vascular inflammation and associated pain	Yes: Several: See Below

This was the only prescription remedy that I have tried that really worked well for me, but its side effects did not let me carry on with my daily routine. I liked this drug because it was able to alleviate my hypersensitivity to light and sound, however it made me feel extremely drowsy. The *triptans*, or selective serotonin receptor agonists are drugs that cause constriction of the vessels in the head in order to reduce the cranial vascular inflammation and thus decrease the source of the pain in migraine. Additional theories have arisen that these drugs are effective because they also act on serotonin receptors in nerve endings. These drugs act by locating serotonin receptors and binding to them to interrupt the chemical process that causes migraine headaches. It sounds complicated, but think of it as placing clay into a keyhole. Even though the key is available, it becomes unable to unlock the door since something has clogged its opening, or the receptor. Common drugs in this category are Glaxo's Imitrex® (and the generic forms of sumatriptan), used to suppress vascular headaches, AstraZeneca's Zomig® (zolmitriptan), used to constrict the vessels in the brain, Glaxo's Amerge® (and the generic forms of naratriptan), and Merck's Maxalt® (and the generic forms of rizatriptan). Common reactions to these drugs are dizziness, drowsiness, muscle and abdominal cramps, nausea, vomiting, diarrhea, hypotension and hypertension, heart palpitations, chest pain, blood clots, possible stroke or cardiac arrest. In that case, someone who has predisposed vascular disorders, hypertension, diabetes, or obesity should not take selective serotonin receptor agonists. Smokers should not take these drugs because it will enhance vasoconstriction already occurring because of smoking. Those who have liver or kidney disease should avoid this medication as well. To increase the benefit of this drug, it is suggested that you take the medication as soon as the symptoms of a migraine headache occur and lay in a dark quiet room for 2 hours after taking the drug. More recently, inhaled and spray formulations of many of these drugs have become available to reduce the time it takes for the drug to have its benefit. As for which of the *triptan* drugs is most effective for treating migraine headaches, several studies have paired these drugs head-to-head, so to speak, and not too surprisingly, the results are mixed depending on which manufacturer sponsors the study. Certain drugs work better for certain individuals, so the results will vary. As to when it is appropriate to seek the aid of a prescription drug, the best advice I could offer is when the over-the-counter and home remedies are ineffective at providing relief and your headaches are becoming more frequent, more intense, or more debilitating, see your doctor and discuss this class of *triptan* drugs.

The table below is a list at the various forms of triptans that have been developed to treat migraine.

The *Triptan* Drugs

Generic Name	Brand Name	Comments
Almotriptan	Axert®	Only *triptan* approved for use in adolescents age 12-17
Frovatriptan	Frova®	Longer lasting and also used for menstrual migraine
Rizatriptan	Maxalt®	A 2nd-generation *triptan* to treat acute migraine
Sumatriptan	Imitrex®	The 1st clinically available *triptan* in US Now available in combination form with naproxen
Zolmitriptan	Zomig®	
Naratriptan	Amerge®	

Chapter 4

Supplemental Relief Remedies

Hot Compresses

How it Works	Comments
Warmth causes relaxation of smooth muscles in blood vessels, also facilitates blood flow to bring medicine to affected area.	Apply warm, wet washcloth to temples, sinus area, and forehead

There are a few theories as to why placing hot compresses on the location of pain helps relieve the pain of a migraine headache. I've learned that when I am in the grips of a migraine, taking Excedrin, and laying in a dark quiet room with a warm washcloth on my eyes and head, helps to relieve my pain the fastest. Applying heat has the ability to slow down muscle contractions therefore placing a hot compresses on the source of pain will slow the smooth muscle contractions of the dilated vessels that are bringing the excessive blood to the head. When the contractions are slowed, the blood is not pushed so forcefully to the brain alleviating a source of migraine pain.

A second theory is that heat increases blood flow to a location. If you were to take a pain reliever such as ibuprofen, acetaminophen, naproxen, or Excedrin, then place a warm washcloth on your eyes, head, or neck, the distribution of the medication to the site of pain is enhanced by the warm compress. Though these theories appear to contradict each other, using a hot compress with a method of pain relief may create combined, synergistic, or more powerful effects.

Cold Compresses

How it Works	Comments
May help dilated blood vessels to shrink to normal size and helps to reduce inflammation.	May work to alternate warm compresses with cold.

It is a matter of opinion as to whether you prefer a hot compress or a cold compress. Personally, with each prolonged migraine attack, I try both. If a hot washcloth doesn't work, I try a cold pack on my head. Cold compresses work well for some people because they cause blood vessels to shrink to their normal size and to slow down the rapid contractions, decreasing the rapid amount of blood flow to your head. Cold compresses will also help relieve the inflammation of the vessels which adds to the pain from migraine headaches. Ice packs and cold compresses can have a pain relieving affect when used for about 15 minutes, causing the area to become numb, relieving the pain. For those who feel that the cold actually makes their pain worsen, remember that cold temperatures cause muscles to contract, and contracting muscles cause the surrounding nerves to feel secondary pain.

Dark and Quiet Room

How it Works	Comments
Eliminating sources of light, sound, and odors helps reduce the intensity of a migraine headache	Use in combination with pain relievers for optimal benefit

Resting in a dark room is encouraged because migraine increases your sensitivity to light. It has been found that the optic nerve inside our brain that controls the function of our eyes and sight is along the same pathway that sends and receives pain receptors in our brains. When experiencing a migraine headache, the light that enters our eyes, increases the activity of the neurons that are active in causing migraine pain. Lying down in a dark room with your eyes shut will prevent the light from further aggravating and intensifying your migraine.

Those who suffer from migraine headaches tend to have sensitivity to sound as well as light. It is suggested that the nerve receptors for sound are located at the center of the brain as well as the serotonin pathways. The serotonin pathways are responsible for the constriction and dilation of the vessels during migraine headaches.

Exercise

How it Works	Comments
Mild non-strenuous exercise may reduce blood pressure, often thought to be a cause for the blood vessel dilation in the head	Best if tried early in the onset. Exercise is not well-tolerated if the migraine pain is severe

Mild, nonstrenuous exercise may be effective at reducing blood pressure, which is believed to be a trigger of the vasodilation process of the blood vessels in the head. If caught early in the onset of head pain, exercise may be effective at thwarting the full blown migraine headache. Many lifelong migraine sufferers claim that adding a daily regimen of walking for 30 minutes is adequate at reducing the frequency of their headaches. For those who are seeking an inexpensive and non-invasive remedy, I suggest starting here – when you have a day that is migraine free. The benefits just may be adequate at reducing the effects of hypertension, a primary trigger of migraine headaches.

Acupuncture

How it Works	Comments
Ancient Chinese treatment that provides reduction of pain and inflammation	Generally more effective at preventing or relieving tension-type headaches

For those seeking a more holistic approach to treating or preventing headaches, acupuncture has been reported to be effective at reducing headaches of the tension variety more so than the migraine variety. It is an old Chinese practice that has been used for thousands of years for the treatment of chronic pain. It is recommended that if you were to choose acupuncture as a way to treat migraines that you follow the regimen of 30 minute, biweekly sessions for 10 weeks.

Chiropractic

How it Works	Comments
Relief of the spinal nerve compression related to subluxations or misalignment of the vertebrae	Generally more effective at prevention than as an acute pain treatment

When the vertebrae found in the neck area of the backbone become misaligned, compression on the base of the brainstem may occur. These spinal misalignments that cause nerve irritation are referred to as subluxations [sub-lux-SAY-shuns] The first two vertebrae are in the cervical region, and are called the C1 and C2 bones. When a C1/C2 subluxation occurs, nerve irritation may develop and in some cases the symptoms of migraine headaches occur. Again, for those seeking a non-invasive, chemical free approach to seeking relief from migraine headaches, seeing a chiropractic physician may provide a solution.

As an athlete and former collegiate softball shortstop, I sought the treatments of a chiropractor to aid in the treatment of my shoulder and upper back strain, as my body was contorted in ways never intended by nature. While my purpose of seeking chiropractic services was not my migraine headaches, I cannot say with any certainty that the frequency of my migraine headaches was reduced while under the care of a chiropractic physician.

Yoga

How it Works	Comments
Relaxation and stress-relief help to reduce blood pressure	Only non-strenuous poses should be used during a migraine episode

Through guided relaxation and stress-relief, some people swear by the benefits of Yoga at preventing, and in some cases providing relief of migraine headache pain. Here the benefits are likely realized by a reduction in the blood pressure. As a precaution, during the grips of a severe migraine headache, Yoga is not recommended.

Head Wraps and Head Bands

How it Works	Comments
Applying direct pressure to the firing nerve cells may deflect or diffuse the pain	May be used in conjunction with hot or cold compresses

One trick that migraine sufferers have used since ancient times to relieve the pain of a migraine headache is applying pressure to the painful area of the head, such as the temples, or binding or wrapping the head with a tight wrap or head band. Some also combine this method with heat or cold, depending on their preference. The reason for this method providing relief in some cases may be due to the applied pressure reducing the firing of pain cells in and around the affected area of the brain. The relief may be temporary, but sufficient to provide a medication-free treatment for relaying pain signals during a migraine attack. If it works, and I intentionally use the word, "if", it provides a benign treatment that may add relief to other strategies, like relaxation or medications.

Good Ol' Fashion Sleep!

How it Works	Comments
Reduces blood pressure, relieves the eyes of light stimuli	Too much sleep can be a migraine trigger

There is nothing quite like quality restorative sleep that works to reset the migraine mechanism, that mechanism that resides within all of us migraine sufferers. When we are tired from over exertion and especially lack of sleep, and our brains need to remain alert at school or work, our stay awake mechanism often includes the body's attempt to raise our blood pressure. As you have heard as a familiar theme in this book, what follows is the dilation of the blood vessels as an attempt to lower the blood pressure, and the inflammation and associated pain follows in the form of a migraine headache. Sleeping off a migraine headache, especially in a dark room, free of scents, filtered of noise, in a temperature that is conducive to sleep, in clothing that is loose and comfortable, is the answer. Be mindful that too much sleep or inconsistent sleep patterns are known to bring about migraine headaches. As a note, a much more comprehensive look at migraine triggers is found in the full version of the *What If It's...* *Migraines* book from Portrait Health Publishing.

Chapter 5

So, where do I start?

The simple answer is, think simplest solution first, but don't waste time. At the earliest sign, and I mean at the very first thought that a migraine headache is lurking, take action. Migraine headaches usually do not start to come on and then just go away on their own. Look at your situation. Are you traveling or in transit? Are you at work or school? Are you still in bed? Is staying at home an option? If you're at work or school, is going home an option? Are you sick and taking medication for another illness? The go-to solution may be totally different based on where you are and what lies ahead in your day. If you have been prescribed a migraine medication, whether a pain-reliever or a vasoconstricting *triptan* drug, and you cannot afford the debilitating pain at school or work, take your medication as soon as possible. If you plan on being at home for the day or are heading home, perhaps an OTC pain reliever is more suitable. As a clinical professional, I would be remiss if I did not include a statement here that you are never alone in caring for yourself. Migraine headaches are very serious, and are not intended to be managed without talking with a medical or clinical professional who knows your health history and is familiar with your medications. As one of the more than 28 million Americans who face the battles of managing migraine, I can tell you that despite a broad background of the physiology, therapies and pharmacology, I rely upon my fellow clinicians to provide me with the answers that have eluded me, and you should do the same with your doctor.

If you would like to share a therapy or remedy, or combination of treatments that works particularly well for you, email us at info@portraithealthpublishing.com. My medical colleagues and I will provide our feedback and keep our followers informed of new information.

References:

1. http://www.mayoclinic.com/health/maois/HQ01575

2. http://emedicine.medscape.com/article/1142556-overview#aw2aab6b2b3aa

3. http://natural-health-alternative.blogspot.com/2010/02/migraines-dilationconstriction-of-blood.html

4. Kees, J.L, Hayes, E.R. & McCuistion, L.E. (2009). *Pharmacology: A nursing process approach* (6th ed.). St. Louis, MO: Mosby.

5. Skidmore-Roth, L., (2008). *Mosby's Nursing Drug Reference.* St. Louis: Mosby.

6. http://www.drugs.com

Appendix

Migraine Triggers App (Answer Key)

If you haven't played the Migraine Triggers App, download it today from iTunes for iPhones or the Android App Store.

Introduction: While migraine headaches may start on their own, there are many avoidable triggers that could bring on a migraine. Most of these common triggers are in the category of food and drink. Test your knowledge in this quiz.

Food and Drink Triggers

1. Of these breakfast beverages, which one should be avoided by somebody who is prone to migraine headaches?

☐ Chai Tea   *No, ginger-containing teas have actually been shown to prevent migraine headaches*

☐ Apple Juice   *No, apples and apple juice are not known as common migraine triggers*

☐ Black Tea   *CORRECT! The tannins in black tea may serve as triggers for migraine* sufferers

☐ Skim Milk   *No, fresh dairy products are on the safe list for migraine sufferers*

2. At a cocktail party, which alcoholic beverage is NOT your best choice?

☐ White Wine   *No, a glass of white wine is generally well tolerated by migraine sufferers*
☐ Vodka   *No, Vodka is a safe choice when consumed slowly and in moderation*
☐ Red Wine   *CORRECT! Red wine is high in tyramines and tannins, two potent migraine triggers.*
☐ Scotch   *No, sipping a glass of Scotch whiskey is generally considered safe for migraine sufferers*

3. Which of these dairy products is considered the safest to those with migraine?

☐ Aged cheese   *No, aged cheese is high in tyramines which are powerful migraine triggers*
☐ Processed cheese   *CORRECT! Processed cheeses are on the safe list of dairy foods*
☐ Sour Cream   *No, aged foods have a higher content of tyramines which could trigger a migraine*
☐ Yogurt   *No, aged foods have a higher content of tyramines which could trigger a migraine*

4. At the sandwich shop, which of these meats is your best choice to top your flatbead to avoid a migraine?

☐ Salami   *No, salami is often high in sodium nitrite, which is a trigger for migraine headaches*
☐ Smoked Ham   *No, smoked meats are high in sodium nitrite, a potent trigger for migraine headaches*
☐ Corned Beef   *No, cured meats contain sodium nitrite, which can trigger a migraine headache*
☐ Chicken Breast   *CORRECT! Fresh, white chicken meat is on the safe list for migraine sufferers*

5. Your sweet tooth is in need of dessert, and you have four choices. Which is not a good choice for migraine sufferers?

☐ Strawberry Jello®   *No, gelatin desserts are safe for migraine sufferers*
☐ Chocolate Ice Cream   *CORRECT! Unfortunately chocolate anything could bring on a migraine headache*
☐ Coffee Cake   *No, unless it contains an aged cheese, coffee cake is considered safe for migraine sufferers*
☐ Ginger Snaps   *No, ginger is actually a spice used to help prevent migraines*

6. Monosodium glutamate (MSG) is a common trigger for migraine. Which does NOT typically contain MSG?

☐ Soy Sauce   *No, most soy sauces contain MSG*
☐ Seasoning Salt   *No, most seasoned salts contain MSG as a flavor enhancer*
☐ White Vinegar   *CORRECT! White wine vinegar is on the safe list of condiments and salad toppers*
☐ Canned Soup   *No, unless the label specifically says otherwise, most canned soups are loaded with MSG*

7. Even many fruits are known to be migraine triggers. What is your best choice among these?

☐ Banana   *No, bananas, especially aged ones, are high in the dreaded tyramines, a known trigger*
☐ Red Globe Grapes   *No, the tannins in the skin and seeds may serve as triggers*
☐ Pear   *CORRECT! Pears and Apples are among your best fruit choices to avoid migraines*
☐ Raisins   *No, aged and dried fruits are high in tyramines, a potent migraine trigger*

8. When deciding on the best sandwich for work or school lunch, what should you avoid?

☐ Peanut Butter & Jelly *CORRECT! Peanuts, and most nuts, contain high amounts of tyramine, a strong trigger*
☐ Fresh Turkey *No, freshly sliced turkey is on the safe list for migraine sufferers*
☐ Fresh Chicken *No, fresh, white poultry meats like chicken breast is safe for migraine sufferers*
☐ Egg Salad *No, hard boiled eggs are generally well-tolerated by migraine sufferers*

9. When tossing a garden salad, which veggie is best left in the crisper if you're a migraine sufferer?

☐ Carrots *No, carrots are on the safe list for foods well tolerated by migraine sufferers*
☐ Tomatoes *No, tomatoes are not known to commonly trigger a migraine headache*
☐ Iceberg Lettuce *No, mainly water in content, iceberg lettuce is a safe salad base for migraine sufferers*
☐ Avocados *CORRECT! Avocados are high in tyramines which are potent migraine triggers*

10. Which bread product is your best choice to avoid a migraine headache?

☐ Cheddar Bread   *No, aged cheeses contain the migraine trigger called tyramine*
☐ Corn Tortilla   *CORRECT! Not only gluten-free, but yeast-free, and on the safe list for migraine*
☐ Sourdough Bread   *No, sourdough breads are high in tyramines which are potent migraine triggers*
☐ Fresh baked Bread   *No, yeasty baked bread products contain the trigger called tyramine*

Physical and Environmental Triggers

Introduction: Not all known triggers to migraine headaches are of the food variety. There are many physical and environmental causes that may trigger a migraine episode. See how you do with these quiz questions:

1. When might a migraine sufferer be most prone to developing a headache?

☐ After a night of Poor Sleep *CORRECT! Lack of quality sleep is one of the most common migraine triggers*
☐ After a 30-minute walk *No, moderate exercise is actually thought to reduce the frequency of headaches*
☐ After a Yoga session *No, relaxation techniques reduce stress and the frequency of headaches*
☐ While listening to soft music *No, soothing sounds tend to reduce stress and blood pressure*

2. Which is an example of a sensory source of hypersensitivity that could trigger a migraine headache?

☐ Wearing Sunglasses *No, UV-protecting sunglasses are often recommended to avoid bright light sensitivity*
☐ Perfumes *CORRECT! The fragrance department in stores should be avoided by migraine sufferers*
☐ Warm Blankets *No, comfortably warm blankets can help you to find a state of relaxation*
☐ Sugary Sweets *No, sweet-tasting foods are not known to trigger migraine headaches*

3. Sudden changes in hormones may lead to a migraine headache. Which is NOT a common hormone trigger?

☐ Premenstrual syndrome   *No, hormone levels change just prior to menstruation*

☐ Stress   *No, cortisol levels due to high stress are known to trigger migraines*

☐ Taking Birth Control Pills   *No, most birth control pills contain hormones*

☐ Taking a B-Vitamin   *CORRECT! The B-Vitamins are not hormones and are used to prevent migraines*

4. A change in barometric pressure may cause the onset of a migraine headache. Which of these natural phenomena is associated with a change in the barometric pressure?

☐ A rainbow   *No, a rainbow is a caused by the diffracting of light through a prism or water droplets*

☐ A thunderstorm   *CORRECT! The sudden pressure change of an approaching storm serves as a trigger*

☐ A sunset   *No, barometric pressure is not changed as light diminishes at sunset*

☐ A full moon   *No, while the moon affects the tides, it does not affect the barometric pressure*

5. Which of these behaviors could bring on a migraine headache when you least expect to have one?

☐ Sleeping in on the weekend *CORRECT! Surprisingly, sleeping more than typical is known to trigger a migraine*

☐ Eating between meals *No, avoiding a state of fasting helps to prevent migraines (Avoid food triggers!)*

☐ Light Exercise *No, typically non-strenuous exercise helps to reduce the frequency of migraines*

☐ Breathing Exercises *No, methods to reduce stress and blood pressure reduce migraine frequency*

6. Which of these physical ailments could trigger a migraine headache?

☐ Dandruff *No, scaling of the dermis of the scalp is not known to trigger a migraine episode*

☐ Toothache *CORRECT! Inflammation of the nerves of the head and oral cavity could be a trigger*

☐ Ankle Sprain *No, typically peripheral pain is not sufficient to serve as a trigger for migraine*

☐ Gout *No, high levels of uric acid associated with gout is not a known migraine trigger*

7. Which mental health disorder is NOT associated with an increased migraine frequency?

- [ ] Depression   *No, depression is associated with an increased tendency for migraine*
- [ ] Anxiety   *No, anxiety is associated with an increased tendency for migraine*
- [ ] Grief   *No, those who are grieving are more prone to migraine*
- [ ] Dementia   *CORRECT! Dementia is not known to be connected to migraines*

8. After a long commute home through the city during rush hour, which of these are NOT considered a trigger to that migraine headache that is developing?

- [ ] Headlight glare   *No, bright and flashing lights are a known migraine trigger*
- [ ] Truck diesel fumes   *No, fumes from hydrocarbon emissions serve as migraine headache triggers*
- [ ] The news on the radio   *CORRECT! Soothing or monotonous sounds are not considered to be migraine triggers*
- [ ] Stopping and starting   *No, jerky motions could not only lead to nausea, but the onset of a migraine headache*

9. Which of these bad moves in a busy day could trigger a migraine?

☐ Skipping Lunch   *CORRECT! Extended periods of fasting during a busy day could trigger a migraine*
☐ Forgetting your wallet   *No, that is just silly.*
☐ Taking time to stretch   *No, just the opposite. Stretching and light exercise could prevent stress*
☐ Taking a flight of stairs   *No, most light exercise helps to avoid the onset of migraine headaches*

10. Sitting in a hot classroom or meeting room is a likely trigger for migraine since:

☐ Heat lowers blood pressure   *No, just the opposite*
☐ Heat raises blood pressure   *CORRECT! In most, temperature increase leads to blood pressure increase*
☐ Low Humidity is a trigger   *No, dry air is not known to be a migraine trigger*
☐ High Oxygen is a trigger   *No, the oxygen content is not known to trigger migraines*